CHAPTER 1: INTRODUCTION TO INTERMITTENT FASTING

What is Intermittent Fasting?

Intermittent fasting has gained significant attention in recent years as a popular approach to weight loss and overall health improvement. But what exactly is intermittent fasting? In this subchapter, we will delve into the concept of intermittent fasting and explore its benefits and essential practices.

Intermittent fasting, in simple terms, is an eating pattern that involves alternating periods of fasting and eating. It is not a diet in the traditional sense but rather a lifestyle choice that focuses on when to eat rather than what to eat. The primary goal of intermittent fasting is to optimize the body's metabolic processes and promote overall well-being.

There are several different methods of intermittent fasting, each with its own variations, but the most common ones include the 16/8 method, where individuals fast for 16 hours and have an eating window of 8 hours, and the 5:2 method, where individuals eat normally for five days a week and restrict their calorie intake on the remaining two days.

The benefits of intermittent fasting extend beyond weight loss. Research suggests that intermittent fasting can improve insulin sensitivity, reduce inflammation, promote cellular repair, and even enhance brain function. It may also help lower the risk of chronic diseases such as diabetes, heart disease, and certain types of cancer.

To effectively practice intermittent fasting, it is crucial to understand the essential practices associated with it. These practices include listening to your body's hunger and fullness cues, staying hydrated, consuming nutrient-dense foods during the eating window, and incorporating regular exercise into your routine. It is also essential to maintain consistency and gradually adapt to the fasting periods to avoid any adverse effects.

It is worth noting that intermittent fasting may not be suitable for everyone. Pregnant or breastfeeding women, individuals with a history of eating disorders, and those with underlying medical conditions should consult with their healthcare provider before embarking on an intermittent fasting journey. In conclusion, intermittent fasting is a flexible and effective approach to improve overall health and achieve weight loss goals. By understanding the concept and adopting the essential practices, anyone can harness the benefits of intermittent fasting and optimize their well-being. So, if you are looking for a dynamic fasting method to improve your health, intermittent fasting may be just the lifestyle change you need.

HISTORY OF INTERMITTENT FASTING

Intermittent fasting is not a new concept; it has been practiced for centuries by various cultures and religions. Understanding the history of intermittent fasting can provide valuable insights into its significance and benefits.

The roots of intermittent fasting can be traced back to ancient civilizations such as the Greeks and Romans. Fasting was seen as a way to cleanse the body and improve mental clarity. Philosophers like Plato and Hippocrates advocated for fasting to enhance overall health and well-being.

Religious practices have also played a significant role in the history of intermittent fasting. Many major religions, including Christianity, Islam, and Buddhism, incorporate fasting as a spiritual discipline. Fasting during specific times or religious holidays has been a tradition for centuries, and it continues to be observed by millions of people worldwide.

One of the most well-known historical figures associated with intermittent fasting is Leonardo da Vinci. He famously practiced a form of fasting called "Bifore," where he would fast for extended periods to enhance his mental focus and creativity. Da Vinci believed that fasting allowed him to tap into higher levels of productivity and imagination.

In recent years, intermittent fasting has gained popularity due to its potential health benefits. Scientific research has shown that intermittent fasting can improve metabolic health, promote weight loss, and increase longevity. This has led to the development of various fasting protocols, such as the 16/8 method, alternate-day fasting, and the 5:2 diet.

Today, intermittent fasting is not only practiced for religious or spiritual reasons but also as a lifestyle choice for improving overall health and well-being. Many celebrities, athletes, and wellness enthusiasts have embraced intermittent fasting and have shared their success stories, further popularizing this approach. Mastering intermittent fasting requires understanding its historical significance and how it has evolved over time. By recognizing the cultural, religious, and scientific foundations of intermittent fasting, individuals can make informed decisions about incorporating it into their lives.

In conclusion, the history of intermittent fasting is a rich tapestry woven with cultural traditions, religious practices, and scientific discoveries. From the ancient Greeks and Romans to modern-day celebrities, intermittent fasting has stood the test of time as a powerful tool for optimizing health and promoting longevity. By delving into its historical roots, we can appreciate the profound impact intermittent fasting has had on human health and well-being throughout the ages.

BENEFITS OF INTERMITTENT FASTING

Intermittent fasting has gained significant popularity in recent years as a powerful tool for optimizing health and achieving weight loss goals. This subchapter explores the numerous benefits of incorporating intermittent fasting into your lifestyle. Regardless of your age, gender, or fitness level, intermittent fasting can offer a wide range of advantages that go beyond just shedding a few pounds.

One of the primary benefits of intermittent fasting is improved insulin sensitivity. By abstaining from food for extended periods, your body becomes more efficient at utilizing insulin, resulting in lower blood sugar levels. This can help prevent the development of type 2 diabetes and reduce the risk of insulin resistance. Additionally, intermittent fasting has been shown to promote autophagy, a cellular process that removes waste material and damaged cells, leading to improved cellular health and longevity.

Another key benefit is enhanced weight loss and fat burning. Intermittent fasting triggers a metabolic switch, forcing your body to tap into its fat stores for energy. During the fasting period, your body depletes its glycogen reserves, and once those are exhausted, it starts burning fat for fuel. This can lead to a significant reduction in body fat and an improvement in body composition.

Furthermore, intermittent fasting has been linked to increased mental clarity and focus. By giving your digestive system a break, your body can redirect energy towards cognitive function. Many individuals report improved concentration, mental sharpness, and better overall brain health when practicing intermittent fasting.

Additionally, intermittent fasting has been found to have positive effects on heart health. It can lower blood pressure, reduce cholesterol levels, and decrease the risk of heart disease. Fasting also promotes the production of human growth hormone (HGH), which plays a crucial role in muscle growth, fat loss, and overall vitality.

Intermittent fasting has also been shown to have anti-inflammatory effects in the body. Chronic inflammation is at the root of many diseases, including arthritis, cardiovascular diseases, and certain types of cancer. By reducing inflammation, intermittent fasting can help prevent and alleviate these conditions, leading to improved overall health.

In conclusion, intermittent fasting offers a multitude of benefits for anyone looking to optimize their health and well-being. From improved insulin sensitivity to enhanced weight loss, increased mental clarity, and reduced inflammation, incorporating intermittent fasting into your lifestyle can have a transformative impact on your overall health. Embrace the power of intermittent fasting and unlock the key to optimal health.

COMMON MYTHS AND MISCONCEPTIONS

When it comes to intermittent fasting, there are several common myths and misconceptions that often lead to confusion and misinformation. In this subchapter, we will debunk these myths and provide you with accurate information to help you understand the true essence of intermittent fasting.

Myth 1: Intermittent fasting is a form of starvation. One of the most prevailing myths surrounding intermittent fasting is that it is synonymous with starvation. This is far from the truth. Intermittent fasting is a deliberate and controlled approach to eating patterns, where you cycle between periods of eating and fasting. It is not about depriving yourself of food; rather, it focuses on optimizing your body's natural mechanisms and promoting overall health.

Myth 2: Intermittent fasting slows down your metabolism. Another misconception is that intermittent fasting slows down your metabolism, making it harder for you to lose weight. Research has shown that intermittent fasting actually helps to increase metabolic rate, improve insulin sensitivity, and enhance fat burning. By giving your body regular periods of fasting, you are allowing it to tap into its fat stores for energy, leading to effective weight loss.

Myth 3: Intermittent fasting leads to muscle loss. Many people believe that intermittent fasting causes muscle loss. However, when done correctly, intermittent fasting can actually help preserve and even increase muscle mass. During fasting periods, your body activates certain cellular pathways that promote muscle preservation. Additionally, when paired with regular resistance exercise, intermittent fasting can lead to significant gains in muscle strength and hypertrophy.

Myth 4: Intermittent fasting is only for weight loss. While weight loss is one of the benefits of intermittent fasting, it is not the sole purpose. Intermittent fasting has been shown to have numerous health benefits, including improved brain function, increased longevity, reduced inflammation, and enhanced cellular repair. It is a holistic approach to health and well-being, aimed at optimizing your body's natural processes.

Myth 5: Intermittent fasting is not suitable for everyone. Contrary to popular belief, intermittent fasting can be practiced by anyone, regardless of age or gender. However, it is important to consult with a healthcare professional before embarking on any fasting regimen, especially if you have pre-existing medical conditions or are taking medication. They can guide you on the most suitable approach and help you tailor it to your individual needs.

In conclusion, intermittent fasting is not a form of starvation, but rather a deliberate and controlled approach to eating patterns. It has numerous benefits beyond weight loss, including improved metabolism, muscle preservation, and overall health optimization. Remember to consult with a healthcare professional before starting any fasting regimen to ensure it is safe and suitable for you.

CHAPTER 2: UNDERSTANDING THE SCIENCE BEHIND INTERMITTENT FASTING

How Intermittent Fasting Affects your Body

Intermittent fasting has gained significant popularity in recent years as an effective approach to weight loss and overall health improvement. But beyond the superficial benefits, how exactly does intermittent fasting affect your body? In this subchapter, we will explore the various ways that this eating pattern can positively impact your overall well-being.

One of the key effects of intermittent fasting is its ability to regulate insulin levels in the body. By abstaining from food for extended periods, your body becomes more insulin sensitive, which means it can better utilize glucose for energy. This can lead to improved blood sugar control and reduced risk of developing insulin resistance, type 2 diabetes, and metabolic syndrome.

Furthermore, intermittent fasting promotes autophagy, a natural cellular cleaning process that helps remove damaged cells and waste products from the body. This process not only aids in detoxification but also plays a crucial role in preventing age-related diseases, such as Alzheimer's and Parkinson's.

Intermittent fasting also has a profound impact on your energy metabolism. When you fast, your body is forced to tap into its fat stores for energy, leading to increased fat burning. This can be particularly beneficial for those looking to shed excess weight or reduce body fat percentage. Additionally, fasting triggers the production of human growth hormone (HGH), which aids in building lean muscle mass and improving athletic performance.

Beyond weight loss and muscle gain, intermittent fasting has been shown to have positive effects on cognitive function and brain health. By promoting the production of brain-derived neurotrophic factor (BDNF), fasting can enhance cognition, improve memory, and protect against neurodegenerative diseases like Alzheimer's and dementia.

Moreover, intermittent fasting can have significant anti-inflammatory effects on the body. Chronic inflammation is linked to various health conditions, including heart disease, cancer, and autoimmune disorders. By reducing inflammation, fasting can help lower the risk of these diseases and promote overall longevity.

While intermittent fasting offers numerous benefits, it is essential to approach it with caution and consult a healthcare professional before embarking on any fasting regimen, especially if you have pre-existing medical conditions or are taking medications.

In conclusion, intermittent fasting is a powerful tool that can positively impact your body in multiple ways. From regulating insulin levels and promoting autophagy to boosting energy metabolism and improving cognitive function, this eating pattern has the potential to optimize your overall health and well-being. However, it is crucial to approach intermittent fasting responsibly and seek guidance from professionals to ensure its safety and effectiveness for your individual needs.

The Role of Insulin in Intermittent Fasting

Intermittent fasting has gained significant popularity in recent years due to its numerous health benefits. One of the key players in this fasting practice is insulin, a hormone that plays a crucial role in regulating our blood sugar levels. Understanding the role of insulin in intermittent fasting is essential for anyone looking to optimize their health through this dietary approach.

Insulin is primarily known for its role in the body's metabolism of carbohydrates. When we consume carbohydrates, our body breaks them down into glucose, which is then released into the bloodstream. In response to this increase in blood glucose, the pancreas releases insulin, which acts as a signal for cells to take up glucose and use it for energy production.

During periods of fasting, when no food is consumed for an extended period, insulin levels decrease significantly. This decrease in insulin allows our body to tap into stored energy reserves, such as glycogen in the liver and fat stored in adipose tissue. As a result, intermittent fasting can promote weight loss and fat burning.

Moreover, intermittent fasting has been shown to improve insulin sensitivity, which is the ability of cells to respond to insulin effectively. Chronically elevated insulin levels, often seen in individuals with insulin resistance or type 2 diabetes, can lead to various health issues, including weight gain, inflammation, and increased risk of chronic diseases.

By practicing intermittent fasting, individuals can give their body a break from constant insulin release, allowing cells to become more sensitive to insulin when it is present. This improved insulin sensitivity can enhance the body's ability to regulate blood sugar levels, leading to better overall metabolic health.

In addition to its effects on weight management and insulin sensitivity, intermittent fasting has also been shown to reduce chronic inflammation, improve brain function, and promote cellular repair and regeneration. These benefits are partly attributed to the role of insulin in intermittent fasting.

In conclusion, understanding the role of insulin in intermittent fasting is vital for anyone looking to optimize their health through this dietary practice. By reducing insulin levels during fasting periods, individuals can promote weight loss, improve insulin sensitivity, and reap numerous other health benefits. Incorporating intermittent fasting into one's lifestyle can be a powerful tool for achieving optimal health and well-being.

IMPACT OF INTERMITTENT FASTING ON WEIGHT LOSS

Intermittent fasting has gained significant popularity in recent years, not only as a tool for weight loss but also for its potential health benefits. In this subchapter, we will explore the impact of intermittent fasting on weight loss and how it can be effectively utilized to achieve optimal results.

Intermittent fasting is an eating pattern that involves cycling between periods of fasting and eating. There are various methods of intermittent fasting, including the 16/8 method, alternate-day fasting, and the 5:2 diet. Regardless of the method chosen, intermittent fasting can have a profound impact on weight loss.

One of the primary ways intermittent fasting aids in weight loss is by promoting a calorie deficit. By restricting the eating window and consuming fewer meals, individuals naturally consume fewer calories overall. This calorie deficit forces the body to tap into its fat stores for energy, leading to weight loss.

Moreover, intermittent fasting can also increase the production of human growth hormone (HGH), which plays a crucial role in fat burning and muscle preservation. This hormone is especially beneficial for those looking to lose weight as it helps preserve lean muscle mass while promoting fat loss.

Additionally, intermittent fasting can improve insulin sensitivity, another vital factor in weight loss. By reducing insulin levels during fasting periods, the body becomes more efficient at utilizing stored fat for energy. This not only aids in weight loss but also reduces the risk of developing insulin resistance and type 2 diabetes.

Furthermore, intermittent fasting has been shown to have a positive impact on metabolism. It can enhance metabolic flexibility, allowing the body to switch between burning glucose and fat more efficiently. This metabolic adaptation can help individuals achieve sustainable weight loss and maintain a healthy weight in the long run.

It is important to note that while intermittent fasting can be an effective tool for weight loss, it should be approached with caution and tailored to individual needs and preferences. It is recommended to consult with a healthcare professional or a registered dietitian before embarking on an intermittent fasting journey, especially for individuals with pre-existing medical conditions.

In conclusion, intermittent fasting can have a significant impact on weight loss by promoting a calorie deficit, increasing HGH production, improving insulin sensitivity, and enhancing metabolic flexibility. By incorporating intermittent fasting into a well-rounded approach to health and wellness, individuals can achieve optimal weight loss results and improve their overall well-being.

Intermittent Fasting and Autophagy

Autophagy, the natural process of cellular self-cleansing and renewal, has gained significant attention in recent years. In this subchapter, we will explore the fascinating relationship between intermittent fasting and autophagy, and how combining these practices can optimize your health and well-being.

Intermittent fasting, as you may already know, is an eating pattern that alternates between periods of fasting and eating. It has been widely recognized for its numerous health benefits, including weight loss, improved insulin sensitivity, and increased energy levels. However, what many people may not be aware of is the powerful link between intermittent fasting and autophagy.

Autophagy, derived from the Greek words for "self" (auto) and "eating" (phagy), refers to the body's ability to recycle and remove damaged or dysfunctional cellular components. During autophagy, the body breaks down unnecessary or malfunctioning proteins, damaged organelles, and other cellular waste, allowing for the regeneration of healthier and more functional cells.

Intermittent fasting triggers autophagy by depriving the body of nutrients for extended periods. When you fast, your body's energy stores are depleted, and it begins to seek alternative fuel sources. As a result, it turns to autophagy to break down and recycle cellular waste, providing the necessary energy and building blocks for cellular repair and rejuvenation.

By incorporating intermittent fasting into your lifestyle, you can enhance the process of autophagy, leading to a myriad of health benefits. Research suggests that autophagy may play a crucial role in preventing age-related diseases, such as neurodegenerative disorders, cardiovascular diseases, and even certain types of cancer. It also supports immune function, helps regulate inflammation, and promotes longevity.

To harness the potential of intermittent fasting and autophagy, it is essential to adopt a balanced approach. Start by gradually increasing the duration of your fasting periods, allowing your body to adjust and adapt. Aim for at least 16 hours of fasting, with an 8-hour eating window, and gradually extend it to 18 or 20 hours if you feel comfortable.

It is also important to prioritize nutrient-dense foods during your eating periods to support cellular repair and optimize autophagy. Include plenty of fresh vegetables, lean proteins, healthy fats, and whole grains in your meals. Avoid processed foods, refined sugars, and excessive carbohydrates, as they may hinder autophagic processes.

In conclusion, intermittent fasting and autophagy are interconnected practices that can revolutionize your health and well-being. By leveraging the power of autophagy through intermittent fasting, you can enhance cellular repair, promote longevity, and reduce the risk of age-related diseases. Embrace these essential practices for optimal health and unlock the potential within you.

CHAPTER 3: DIFFERENT METHODS OF INTERMITTENT FASTING

The 16/8 Method: Time-restricted Eating

One of the most popular and effective approaches to intermittent fasting is the 16/8 method, also known as time-restricted eating. This method involves restricting you're eating window to 8 hours and fasting for the remaining 16 hours of the day. This approach is simple yet powerful, making it an excellent choice for anyone looking to improve their health and achieve their wellness goals.

The concept behind the 16/8 method is rooted in our body's natural circadian rhythm. Our bodies are designed to function optimally when we align our eating patterns with daylight hours. By eating during a specific window and fasting for the rest of the day, we can synchronize our internal clock, leading to a range of health benefits.

One of the primary advantages of the 16/8 method is its ability to promote weight loss. By limiting the time frame in which you consume food, you naturally reduce your caloric intake. Additionally, when your body is in a fasting state, it switches from burning glucose for energy to burning stored fat. This can lead to significant fat loss over time.

Beyond weight loss, time-restricted eating has been shown to improve several other aspects of health. Studies have found that this method can enhance insulin sensitivity, lower blood sugar levels, and reduce inflammation in the body. It may also have positive effects on brain health, as fasting has been linked to improved cognitive function and a reduced risk of neurodegenerative diseases like Alzheimer's.

Implementing the 16/8 method is relatively straightforward. Simply choose an 8-hour window during the day when you will consume all your meals, and fast for the remaining 16 hours. Many people find it easiest to skip breakfast and have their first meal around midday, then finish eating by early evening. However, you can adjust the timing to fit your schedule and preferences.

As with any dietary change, it's essential to listen to your body and make adjustments as needed. If you find it challenging to adhere to an 8-hour eating window initially, you can start with a wider window and gradually narrow it down. It's also crucial to prioritize nutrient-dense foods during your eating window to ensure you're getting all the necessary vitamins and minerals.

The 16/8 method of time-restricted eating is a fantastic tool for anyone looking to optimize their health. Whether your goal is weight loss, improved metabolic function, or enhanced cognitive performance, this approach can help you achieve it. By aligning your eating patterns with your body's natural rhythm, you'll unlock a range of benefits and take a significant step towards mastering intermittent fasting.

THE 5:2 METHOD: CALORIE RESTRICTION

If you're looking for an effective and flexible way to practice intermittent fasting, the 5:2 method might be just what you need. This approach, also known as the Fast Diet, involves restricting your calorie intake for two non-consecutive days of the week while eating normally for the remaining five days. In "Mastering Intermittent Fasting: Essential Practices for Optimal Health," we delve into the details of this popular technique and how it can benefit anyone, regardless of their health goals or lifestyle.

Calorie restriction has long been associated with numerous health benefits, including weight loss, improved insulin sensitivity, reduced inflammation, and even longevity. The 5:2 method takes advantage of these advantages while offering a more sustainable and manageable approach than traditional daily fasting. By only restricting calories on two days of the week, you can easily fit intermittent fasting into your busy schedule without feeling deprived or overwhelmed.

One of the key aspects of the 5:2 method is the flexibility it provides. You have the freedom to choose which days you want to fast, allowing you to work around social events, family gatherings, or any other commitments. This flexibility makes it easier to adhere to the fasting schedule, increasing your chances of long-term success.

During the two fasting days, men typically consume around 600 calories, while women consume about 500 calories. These calories can be spread throughout the day or consumed in one or two meals, depending on your preference. It's important to focus on nutrient-dense foods during your fasting days to ensure you're getting the necessary vitamins and minerals.

On the non-fasting days, you can eat normally, which means there are no strict restrictions on what or how much you can consume. However, it's important to maintain a balanced and healthy diet to maximize the benefits of intermittent fasting. By combining the 5:2 method with nutritious eating habits, you can achieve optimal results in terms of weight loss, improved energy levels, and overall well-being.

Whether you're looking to shed a few pounds, improve your metabolic health, or simply want to experience the numerous benefits of intermittent fasting, the 5:2 method is an excellent choice. It provides a flexible and sustainable approach to calorie restriction, making it suitable for anyone seeking to optimize their health. Dive into "Mastering Intermittent Fasting: Essential Practices for Optimal Health" and learn how to incorporate the 5:2 method into your life to achieve your health goals.

Alternate Day Fasting

In the quest for optimal health and well-being, intermittent fasting has emerged as a powerful tool. It offers a flexible and sustainable approach to weight loss, improved metabolic health, increased energy levels, and even longevity. Among the various intermittent fasting methods, Alternate Day Fasting (ADF) stands out as a popular and effective approach.

ADF involves alternating between periods of fasting and feasting. It typically consists of a fasting day, during which calorie intake is severely restricted, followed by a day of normal eating. This cycle is repeated throughout the week or month, depending on individual preferences and goals.

One of the key benefits of ADF is its simplicity. Unlike other fasting protocols that require meticulous tracking and planning, ADF offers a more straightforward approach. On fasting days, individuals consume a limited amount of calories, usually around 500-600 calories, or completely abstain from food. On feasting days, there are no restrictions on food intake, allowing for a more intuitive approach to eating.

ADF has been shown to have numerous health benefits. Research suggests that it can promote weight loss by reducing overall calorie intake. By alternating between fasting and feasting, ADF helps create a calorie deficit, leading to fat loss over time. Additionally, ADF can improve insulin sensitivity, lower inflammation, and enhance cellular repair mechanisms, which are crucial for overall health and disease prevention.

Another advantage of ADF is its potential to improve adherence to a fasting regimen. Many individuals find it easier to commit to fasting every other day, rather than following a daily fasting routine. ADF offers flexibility, allowing individuals to plan their fasting and feasting days based on their schedule and preferences.

However, ADF might not be suitable for everyone. It is important to listen to your body and adjust the fasting schedule accordingly. Some individuals may find it challenging to consume a limited number of calories on fasting days, while others may experience excessive hunger or fatigue. It is crucial to prioritize nutrient-dense foods on feasting days to ensure adequate nourishment.

In conclusion, Alternate Day Fasting is an effective and flexible approach to intermittent fasting. It offers a simple and sustainable way to achieve weight loss, improve metabolic health, and promote overall well-being. However, it is essential to personalize the fasting schedule and listen to your body's needs. With proper guidance and adherence, ADF can be a valuable tool in mastering intermittent fasting and optimizing your health.

EXTENDED FASTING: 24 HOURS OR MORE

In the world of intermittent fasting, extended fasting has gained significant attention for its potential health benefits and weight loss effects. While fasting for shorter periods, such as 16-20 hours, can be beneficial, extended fasting of 24 hours or more takes the benefits to a whole new level.

Extended fasting involves abstaining from food for a longer period, typically 24 hours or more. This practice allows the body to enter a state of ketosis, where it begins to burn stored fat for energy instead of relying on glucose from food. As a result, extended fasting can be an effective strategy for weight loss, as it helps the body tap into its fat reserves.

But weight loss is just the tip of the iceberg when it comes to the benefits of extended fasting. Research has shown that it can have a profound impact on various aspects of our health. One of the most notable benefits is its ability to promote autophagy, a natural process that helps the body cleanse and repair damaged cells. During an extended fast, the body triggers autophagy to break down and recycle old or dysfunctional cells, leading to rejuvenation and improved cellular function.

Moreover, extended fasting has been shown to improve insulin sensitivity and regulate blood sugar levels. By giving the body a break from constant food intake, it allows insulin levels to drop, which in turn enhances the body's ability to metabolize glucose effectively. This can be especially beneficial for individuals with conditions like type 2 diabetes or insulin resistance.

Additionally, extended fasting has been linked to improved brain health. Studies have shown that fasting can enhance cognitive function, improve focus and concentration, and even protect against neurodegenerative diseases like Alzheimer's and Parkinson's.

While extended fasting can offer numerous health benefits, it is crucial to approach it with caution and consult a healthcare professional if you have any underlying health conditions. It is also important to listen to your body and break the fast if you experience severe discomfort or adverse effects.

In conclusion, extended fasting of 24 hours or more can be a powerful tool for optimizing health and achieving weight loss goals. By promoting autophagy, improving insulin sensitivity, and enhancing brain health, this practice offers a range of benefits that go beyond mere weight management. However, it is important to approach extended fasting with knowledge and care, ensuring it aligns with your individual health needs and goals.

CHAPTER 4: PREPARING FOR INTERMITTENT FASTING

Consulting with a Healthcare Professional

Intermittent fasting has gained significant popularity in recent years, with many claiming its numerous health benefits. However, before embarking on any fasting regimen, it is essential to consult with a healthcare professional. This subchapter will emphasize the importance of seeking medical advice and provide guidance on how to approach the subject with your healthcare provider.

Intermittent fasting involves alternating periods of eating and fasting, which can have a profound impact on your body and overall well-being. While this approach to eating has shown promising results for weight loss, improved metabolism, and increased energy levels, it may not be suitable for everyone. Consulting with a healthcare professional is crucial to ensure that intermittent fasting aligns with your specific health needs and goals.

When discussing intermittent fasting with your healthcare provider, it is essential to provide them with a comprehensive medical history. This includes any pre-existing conditions, medications, allergies, or previous experiences with fasting. Armed with this information, your healthcare professional can assess whether intermittent fasting is a safe and viable option for you.

Additionally, your healthcare provider can help tailor an intermittent fasting plan that suits your individual needs. They can provide guidance on the duration and frequency of fasting periods, as well as suggest modifications to accommodate any underlying health conditions. If you are currently on medication, your healthcare provider can also advise on how to adjust your medication schedule during fasting periods.

Furthermore, consulting with a healthcare professional can help identify any potential risks or complications associated with intermittent fasting. They can assess whether you have any nutritional deficiencies or imbalances that may need addressing before starting a fasting regimen. Your healthcare provider can also monitor your progress and make any necessary adjustments to ensure optimal health and well-being.

Remember, it is essential to approach intermittent fasting as a collaborative effort between you and your healthcare provider. Open and honest communication is key, as it allows your healthcare professional to provide the best possible guidance and support throughout your fasting journey.

In conclusion, consulting with a healthcare professional before embarking on an intermittent fasting regimen is crucial for anyone considering this approach to eating. By seeking medical advice, you can ensure that intermittent fasting aligns with your specific health needs and goals. Your healthcare provider can tailor a fasting plan, address any potential risks or complications, and provide ongoing support to help you achieve optimal health and well-being. Remember, your health should always be a top priority, and consulting with a healthcare professional is an essential step towards mastering intermittent fasting.

ASSESSING YOUR CURRENT EATING HABITS

When embarking on a journey towards intermittent fasting, it is crucial to assess your current eating habits. Understanding your existing patterns and behaviours will allow you to make informed decisions and tailor your fasting regimen to suit your needs.

Take a moment to reflect on your typical eating schedule. Do you find yourself snacking throughout the day or indulging in large meals late at night? Are you consuming a balanced and nutritious diet, or do you rely heavily on processed foods and sugary treats? Assessing these aspects of your eating habits will help you identify areas for improvement and set realistic goals for your intermittent fasting journey.

Start by keeping a food diary for a week. Record everything you eat and drink, including portion sizes and the time of consumption. This will provide a comprehensive overview of your current eating habits and patterns. Be honest with yourself and refrain from judgment – the purpose of this exercise is to gather information, not to criticize.

Once you have a clear understanding of your eating habits, it's time to evaluate the nutritional value of your diet. Are you consuming enough fruits, vegetables, lean proteins, and whole grains? Or are your meals predominantly composed of processed and fast foods? Consider consulting a nutritionist or dietician to assess your current nutrient intake and make recommendations for improvement.

Additionally, pay attention to your emotional relationship with food. Do you often turn to food for comfort or stress relief? Are you prone to emotional eating? Identifying these patterns will help you develop strategies to address them during your intermittent fasting journey.

Lastly, evaluate your current meal timing. Do you have a consistent eating schedule, or do you eat whenever you feel hungry? Assessing your meal timing will allow you to determine the most suitable fasting window for your lifestyle and preferences.

Remember, assessing your current eating habits is not about shame or guilt; it's about gaining awareness and making positive changes. Armed with this knowledge, you can create a personalized intermittent fasting plan that aligns with your goals and sets you up for success on your journey towards optimal health.

In the upcoming chapters, we will delve deeper into the various intermittent fasting protocols and provide practical tips for implementing them effectively. Get ready to embrace dynamic fasting and unlock the incredible benefits it holds for your overall well-being.

Setting Realistic Goals

In the journey towards achieving optimal health through intermittent fasting, setting realistic goals is crucial. It is important for anyone embarking on this transformative lifestyle to understand that the path to success is not a quick fix, but rather a sustainable and long-term commitment. This subchapter will explore the significance of setting realistic goals and provide essential practices to help you along your intermittent fasting journey

When it comes to intermittent fasting, it is essential to set realistic goals that align with your individual needs, lifestyle, and health objectives. Avoid setting overly ambitious goals that may lead to frustration and disappointment. Instead, focus on attainable milestones that can be achieved gradually over time.

One important practice for setting realistic goals is to assess your current health status and determine what improvements you would like to make. Are you looking to lose weight, lower your blood sugar levels, improve your cardiovascular health, or simply increase your overall well-being? By identifying your specific objectives, you can tailor your intermittent fasting plan to suit your needs.

Another crucial aspect of setting realistic goals is to consider your daily routine and lifestyle. Intermittent fasting can be integrated seamlessly into various schedules, but it is important to choose a fasting window that is practical for you. For instance, if you have a busy work schedule, it might be more realistic to start with a 16:8 fasting schedule, where you fast for 16 hours and have an 8-hour eating window.

Moreover, it is vital to track and monitor your progress as you work towards your goals. Keep a journal or use a fasting app to record your fasting periods, meals, and any changes you notice in your health. This will not only help you stay accountable but also allow you to make adjustments if needed.

Finally, remember to celebrate your achievements along the way. Setting realistic goals means acknowledging and appreciating the small victories. Whether it's losing a few pounds, feeling more energized, or experiencing improved mental clarity, celebrate these milestones and use them as motivation to continue your intermittent fasting journey.

In conclusion, setting realistic goals is an integral part

of mastering intermittent fasting. By assessing your health objectives, considering your lifestyle, tracking your progress, and celebrating achievements, you can create a sustainable and effective intermittent fasting plan tailored to your individual needs. Remember that intermittent fasting is a journey, and by setting realistic goals, you are laying the foundation for long-term success and optimal health.

BUILDING A SUPPORT SYSTEM

In the journey towards mastering intermittent fasting, one crucial aspect that often gets overlooked is the importance of building a strong support system. Embarking on this lifestyle change can be challenging and having a network of people who understand and support your goals can make all the difference. Whether you are just starting out or have been practicing intermittent fasting for a while, surrounding yourself with like-minded individuals can provide invaluable motivation, accountability, and guidance.

First and foremost, it is essential to educate your immediate family and close friends about intermittent fasting and its benefits. Explaining your reasons for adopting this lifestyle can help them understand your commitment and encourage their support. Share with them the scientific research behind intermittent fasting, highlighting its positive impact on health, weight loss, and overall well-being. By involving your loved ones in your journey, you create an environment that fosters encouragement and understanding.

Aside from your personal circle, it is also crucial to seek out communities and groups that specialize in intermittent fasting. Online forums, social media groups, and local meetups are excellent platforms to connect with individuals who share similar goals and challenges. Engaging in discussions, asking questions, and sharing experiences can provide you with a wealth of knowledge and support. Additionally, participating in these communities can help you stay motivated and committed to your intermittent fasting practice.

Consider finding an accountability partner who is also on the intermittent fasting journey. This person can be a friend, co-worker, or even someone you met through an online community. Regular check-ins, sharing progress, and discussing challenges can create a sense of camaraderie and keep you on track. Having someone who understands the ups and downs of intermittent fasting can be incredibly motivating during moments of self-doubt or difficulty.

In addition to personal connections, seeking professional guidance can be immensely beneficial. Consulting a registered dietitian or a nutritionist who specializes in intermittent fasting can provide you with personalized advice and guidance tailored to your specific needs. They can help you navigate through potential hurdles, create a customized meal plan, and ensure that you are meeting your nutritional requirements while practicing intermittent fasting.

Remember, building a support system is not just about receiving support; it is also about giving support. By sharing your experiences, knowledge, and successes with others, you become an inspiration to those around you. Your journey can inspire others to embark on their own intermittent fasting practice, creating a ripple effect of positive change within your community.

In conclusion, building a support system is an integral part of mastering intermittent fasting. Surrounding yourself with individuals who understand and support your goals can provide the motivation, accountability, and guidance needed for success. Educate your loved ones, seek out communities, find an accountability partner, and consider consulting a professional to create a robust support system that will propel you towards optimal health through intermittent fasting.

CHAPTER 5: ESSENTIAL PRACTICES FOR SUCCESSFUL INTERMITTENT FASTING

Choosing Nutrient-Dense Foods

When it comes to practicing intermittent fasting, one of the most crucial aspects is selecting nutrient-dense foods. Nutrient-dense foods not only provide your body with the essential vitamins and minerals it needs for optimal health, but they also help to promote satiety and sustain energy levels throughout the fasting period.

So, what exactly are nutrient-dense foods? These are foods that are rich in nutrients relative to their calorie content. They are typically whole, unprocessed foods that offer a wide range of vitamins, minerals, and antioxidants. By incorporating these foods into your intermittent fasting routine, you can ensure that your body receives the necessary nourishment it needs during the fasting and feeding windows.

Fruits and vegetables should be the cornerstone of your nutrient-dense diet. They are packed with vitamins, minerals, and fibre, which not only promote overall health but also aid in digestion and weight management. Try to include a variety of colours in your diet, as different fruits and vegetables offer different nutrients. Leafy greens, berries, citrus fruits, and cruciferous vegetables are particularly nutrient-dense options.

Lean proteins are another crucial component of a nutrient-dense diet. They provide essential amino acids for muscle repair and growth. opt for sources like skinless poultry, fish, eggs, tofu, and legumes to meet your protein needs while keeping calorie intake in check.

Whole grains are an excellent source of complex carbohydrates and fibre. They provide a slow release of energy, keeping you feeling full and satisfied for longer periods. Choose options like quinoa, brown rice, whole wheat bread, and oats to increase your intake of nutrient-dense grains.

Healthy fats, such as avocados, nuts, seeds, and olive oil, are vital for a balanced diet. They help with nutrient absorption and provide satiety. However, remember to consume them in moderation, as they are also caloriedense.

Lastly, it is essential to avoid or limit highly processed and sugary foods. These items are often devoid of nutrients and can lead to weight gain and various health issues. Instead, opt for whole, natural foods whenever possible.

By choosing nutrient-dense foods, you can optimize your intermittent fasting journey and promote overall health and well-being. Remember to incorporate a wide variety of fruits, vegetables, lean proteins, whole grains, and healthy fats into your meals. Your body will thank you for the nourishment it receives during both fasting and feeding periods.

HYDRATION AND INTERMITTENT FASTING

In the realm of intermittent fasting, the importance of hydration cannot be overstated. While it may seem like a simple concept, staying adequately hydrated during periods of fasting is crucial for maintaining optimal health and reaping the full benefits of this powerful lifestyle practice. In this subchapter, we will explore the significance of hydration during intermittent fasting and provide essential practices to ensure you stay wellhydrated on your fasting journey.

Water is essential for our bodies to function properly, and this becomes even more critical during fasting periods. When we fast, our bodies enter a state of ketosis, where fat stores are broken down for energy. This process produces waste products that need to be flushed out, making hydration essential for efficient detoxification. Additionally, staying hydrated helps to curb hunger pangs, reduce cravings, and maintain energy levels throughout the fasting period.

One of the key challenges of intermittent fasting is maintaining hydration without breaking the fast. While it may be tempting to reach for a glass of juice or a caffeinated beverage, these can disrupt the fasting state and hinder the desired metabolic benefits. Instead, opt for water as your primary source of hydration. Plain water is calorie-free and will not interfere with the fasting process.

To enhance hydration during fasting, consider adding a pinch of sea salt or a squeeze of lemon to your water. Sea salt replenishes electrolytes, which can become imbalanced during fasting, while lemon provides a refreshing taste and supports digestion. Herbal teas and infused water are also excellent hydrating options, as long as they are free from additives or sweeteners.

Timing your hydration is also crucial. During the eating window, prioritize drinking enough water to meet your daily hydration needs. This will ensure that your body has a sufficient supply of water to support all its functions during the fasting period. However, be mindful of excessive water consumption just before the fasting window begins, as it may lead to frequent bathroom breaks during the fast.

In conclusion, staying hydrated is a vital component of successful intermittent fasting. By prioritizing water intake, avoiding caloric beverages, and adding electrolyte-rich additions, you can maintain optimal hydration levels during fasting periods. Remember, the benefits of intermittent fasting are amplified when coupled with proper hydration, so drink up and savour the transformative effects on your health and well-being.

Managing Hunger and Cravings

Hunger and cravings are common challenges that individuals face when practicing intermittent fasting. The urge to eat can be overpowering, making it difficult to adhere to fasting schedules and achieve the desired health benefits. However, with effective strategies and mindful practices, managing hunger and cravings can become easier, enabling individuals to thrive in their intermittent fasting journey.

One of the essential practices for managing hunger and cravings is to ensure a balanced and nutrient-dense diet during the eating window. Consuming whole foods that are rich in fibre, proteins, and healthy fats can help promote satiety and prevent excessive hunger. Including plenty of vegetables, lean proteins, nuts, and seeds in meals can provide the body with the necessary nutrients to stay satisfied for longer periods.

Another key strategy is to stay hydrated throughout the fasting and eating windows. Drinking an adequate amount of water helps curb hunger pangs and can also help differentiate between true hunger and thirst. Additionally, herbal teas or infusions can be consumed to enhance the feeling of fullness and provide a pleasant flavour experience during fasting periods.

Mindfulness techniques can also be powerful tools in managing hunger and cravings. Paying attention to bodily cues and being aware of emotional triggers can help individuals differentiate between actual hunger and emotional cravings. Engaging in activities such as meditation or deep breathing exercises can also help reduce stress levels and minimize the likelihood of stress-induced eating.

Furthermore, individuals can experiment with different fasting schedules to find the one that best suits their needs and helps manage hunger effectively. Some people may find that shorter fasting windows work better for them, while others may thrive with longer fasting periods. It is important to listen to the body and make adjustments as necessary to optimize the fasting experience.

Lastly, seeking support from the intermittent fasting community or a healthcare professional can provide valuable guidance and encouragement. Sharing experiences and learning from others who have successfully managed hunger and cravings can be motivating and offer practical tips for overcoming challenges.

By implementing these essential practices and adopting a mindful approach, anyone can effectively manage hunger and cravings during intermittent fasting. With time and practice, individuals can develop a healthier relationship with food, achieve optimal health, and experience the numerous benefits that intermittent fasting has to offer.

INCORPORATING EXERCISE INTO YOUR FASTING ROUTINE

Exercise is an essential component of a healthy lifestyle, and when combined with intermittent fasting, it can amplify the benefits of both practices. Engaging in physical activity while fasting can help boost your metabolism, promote fat burning, and enhance overall health and well-being. In this subchapter, we will explore various ways to incorporate exercise into your fasting routine, ensuring that you make the most out of both practices.

First and foremost, it is essential to listen to your body and choose an exercise routine that suits your fitness level and fasting goals. If you are new to fasting or exercise, start with low-intensity activities such as walking, yoga, or light resistance training. As your body adapts and becomes more comfortable with fasting, gradually increase the intensity and duration of your workouts.

One popular approach to exercising during fasting is to engage in fasted cardio. This involves performing cardiovascular exercises, such as jogging or cycling, on an empty stomach. When you exercise in a fasted state, your body primarily relies on stored fat as a source of fuel, leading to increased fat burning and weight loss. However, it is important to stay hydrated and listen to your body's signals to avoid overexertion.

Strength training is another excellent option to incorporate into your fasting routine. By lifting weights or engaging in resistance exercises, you can build lean muscle mass, improve your metabolism, and promote fat loss. It is recommended to perform strength training exercises either before breaking your fast or during your eating window to provide your body with the necessary nutrients for muscle repair and growth.

If you prefer a more dynamic and challenging workout, consider high-intensity interval training (HIIT). HIIT involves short bursts of intense exercise followed by brief periods of rest. This type of workout can be extremely effective for fat burning and improving cardiovascular fitness. However, it is crucial to pay attention to your body's limits and gradually increase the intensity and duration of your HIIT sessions.

Remember to prioritize rest and recovery as well. Fasting combined with exercise can put additional stress on your body, so make sure to allow yourself enough time to rest and rejuvenate. Listen to your body's signals and adjust your exercise routine, accordingly, ensuring you strike a balance between pushing yourself and taking care of your overall well-being.

Incorporating exercise into your fasting routine can be a powerful way to optimize your health and fitness goals. Experiment with different types of workouts, find what works best for you, and enjoy the synergistic benefits of intermittent fasting and exercise.

CHAPTER 6: OVERCOMING COMMON CHALLENGES IN INTERMITTENT FASTING

Dealing with Social Situations and Peer Pressure

In today's society, social situations and peer pressure can pose significant challenges when it comes to maintaining a healthy lifestyle and sticking to your intermittent fasting routine. Whether you are new to intermittent fasting or have been practicing it for a while, it is crucial to develop strategies to navigate these situations without compromising your health goals.

One of the most common social situations that can derail your intermittent fasting progress is dining out with friends or family. It can be tempting to give in to peer pressure and indulge in unhealthy food choices. However, with a few simple strategies, you can stay on track while still enjoying social gatherings. Firstly, it is essential to communicate your dietary preferences and goals with your companions. Let them know about your intermittent fasting routine and why it is important to you.

This open communication will help them understand and respect your choices. Secondly, be proactive in selecting restaurants that offer healthy options or customizable meals. Research the menu beforehand and choose meals that align with your fasting window and dietary requirements. Additionally, consider intermittent fasting-friendly alternatives, such as having a small snack before the outing to avoid excessive hunger and making impulsive food choices.

Another social situation that can be challenging is attending parties or events where food and drinks are abundant. Peer pressure can be strong, but it is crucial to stay focused on your health goals. One effective strategy is to bring your own intermittent fasting-friendly dish to share. This way, you can ensure there is at least one healthy option available to you. Additionally, practice mindful eating by listening to your body's hunger and fullness cues. Avoid mindless snacking and instead focus on enjoying the company and engaging in non-food related activities

It is also important to establish a support system to help you deal with peer pressure and stay motivated. Surround yourself with like-minded individuals who understand and support your intermittent fasting journey. Joining online communities or finding an accountability partner can provide the necessary encouragement and guidance when facing challenging social situations.

Remember, intermittent fasting is a personal choice, and it is essential to prioritize your health and well-being above societal pressures. By implementing these strategies and staying committed to your goals, you can successfully navigate social situations and peer pressure while maintaining optimal health through intermittent fasting.

ADDRESSING PLATEAUS AND WEIGHT LOSS RESISTANCE

Plateaus and weight loss resistance can be frustrating and demotivating, especially when you have been diligently following an intermittent fasting regimen. However, it's important to understand that hitting a plateau is a normal part of the weight loss journey, and there are effective strategies to overcome it. In this subchapter, we will explore various techniques to address plateaus and weight loss resistance, allowing you to continue making progress towards your goals.

One common reason for plateaus is the body's natural adaptation to a lower calorie intake and increased metabolic efficiency. Over time, your body may adjust to your new eating pattern, causing weight loss to slow down or come to a halt. To overcome this, it is crucial to introduce periodic variations in your fasting routine. This could involve altering your fasting and feeding windows, incorporating longer fasting periods, or experimenting with different types of fasting such as alternate-day fasting or 24-hour fasting.

Another factor that can contribute to weight loss resistance is stress. Chronic stress can lead to hormonal imbalances, specifically elevated cortisol levels, which can hinder weight loss efforts. Therefore, it is essential to find effective stress management techniques, such as meditation, yoga, or engaging in activities you enjoy. Additionally, ensuring adequate sleep and rest is crucial for optimizing your body's ability to lose weight.

Dietary factors also play a significant role in overcoming plateaus and weight loss resistance. It may be helpful to reassess your macronutrient ratios and ensure you are consuming a balanced diet with sufficient protein, healthy fats, and complex carbohydrates. Incorporating nutrient-dense foods, such as fruits, vegetables, and lean proteins, can provide essential vitamins and minerals while promoting satiety.

In some cases, underlying medical conditions or medications may contribute to weight loss resistance. It is advisable to consult with a healthcare professional to rule out any underlying issues that might be hindering your progress. They can provide tailored advice and help you navigate through any potential obstacles.

Lastly, maintaining a positive mindset and staying patient is crucial when addressing plateaus and weight loss resistance. Remember that weight loss is not always linear, and your body may need time to adapt and readjust. Celebrate non-scale victories, such as increased energy levels or improved mental clarity, as they indicate progress towards optimal health.

By implementing these strategies and staying committed to your intermittent fasting journey, you can overcome plateaus and weight loss resistance, ultimately achieving your health and wellness goals. Stay determined, stay focused, and embrace the journey towards mastering intermittent fasting.

Coping with Emotional Eating

Emotional eating is a common challenge that many people face when trying to adopt a healthier lifestyle, especially during intermittent fasting. It refers to the tendency of turning to food for comfort or as a coping mechanism in response to emotional triggers such as stress, sadness, boredom, or anxiety.

Understanding and managing emotional eating is crucial to maintaining a successful intermittent fasting practice and achieving optimal health.

Recognizing Emotional Eating Patterns

The first step in coping with emotional eating is to become aware of your own patterns. Take a moment to reflect on your eating habits and identify any emotional triggers that lead you to indulge in unhealthy food choices. It could be a long day at work, a fight with a loved one, or simply feeling lonely. By recognizing these triggers, you can begin to take control of your response to them.

Finding Alternative Coping Strategies

Once you have identified your emotional triggers, it's important to find alternative coping strategies that don't involve food. Engaging in activities that bring you joy and help you relax can be incredibly beneficial. This could include practicing mindfulness or meditation, going for a walk in nature, listening to music, or engaging in a hobby you enjoy. By finding healthier ways to manage your emotions, you can break the cycle of emotional eating.

Building a Support Network

Having a support network is crucial when it comes to coping with emotional eating. Surrounding yourself with people who understand your goals and can provide encouragement and accountability can make a big difference. Consider joining an intermittent fasting support group online or in your community where you can share experiences, seek advice, and find inspiration from others on the same journey.

Mindful Eating Practices

Practicing mindful eating can also help in coping with emotional eating. Mindful eating involves paying attention to your body's hunger and fullness cues, as well as savouring each bite of food. By slowing down and fully engaging with your meals, you can better connect with your body's needs and prevent mindless eating in response to emotions.

Seeking Professional Help

If emotional eating becomes a persistent challenge that is difficult to overcome on your own, it may be beneficial to seek professional help. A therapist or counsellor can provide guidance and support in navigating emotional triggers and developing healthier coping mechanisms. They can also help address any underlying emotional issues that may be contributing to emotional eating.

Remember, coping with emotional eating is a journey that takes time and patience. By being mindful of your triggers, finding alternative coping strategies, building a support network, practicing mindful eating, and seeking professional help if needed, you can overcome emotional eating and cultivate a healthier relationship with food during your intermittent fasting journey.

MANAGING SIDE EFFECTS OF INTERMITTENT FASTING

Intermittent fasting has gained immense popularity in recent years as a powerful tool for weight loss, improved metabolic health, and longevity. However, like any dietary practice, it is essential to be aware of and manage potential side effects that may arise during the fasting period. By understanding and addressing these side effects, you can ensure a smoother and more enjoyable intermittent fasting journey.

One common side effect of intermittent fasting is hunger pangs. As your body adjusts to the new eating pattern, it is natural to experience increased hunger during the fasting hours. To manage this, it is crucial to stay hydrated by drinking plenty of water, herbal teas, or low-calorie beverages. These can help suppress hunger and keep you feeling satisfied. Additionally, consuming high-fibre foods during your eating window can promote a feeling of fullness.

Another side effect that some individuals may experience is low energy levels or fatigue. This can occur as your body adapts to using stored fat as an energy source instead of carbohydrates. To combat this, ensure you are consuming a balanced diet during your eating window, including nutrient-dense foods such as lean proteins, whole grains, fruits, and vegetables. Additionally, getting enough sleep and incorporating regular exercise can improve energy levels and overall well-being.

Some people may also encounter digestive issues, such as constipation or diarrhoea, during intermittent fasting. This can be attributed to changes in the gut microbiome and altered eating patterns. To alleviate these symptoms, it is important to include an adequate amount of dietary fibre in your meals and stay hydrated. Fibre-rich foods, such as whole grains, legumes, and vegetables, can promote healthy digestion and regular bowel movements.

Lastly, it is crucial to monitor your mental and emotional well-being while practicing intermittent fasting. Some individuals may experience increased irritability, mood swings, or difficulty concentrating. These changes can be attributed to hunger or fluctuations in blood sugar levels. To manage these side effects, prioritize self-care activities such as meditation, yoga, or spending time in nature. These practices can help reduce stress levels and improve overall mental well-being.

In conclusion, managing side effects is an essential aspect of mastering intermittent fasting. By understanding common issues such as hunger pangs, low energy levels, digestive issues, and mood changes, you can take proactive steps to mitigate these effects. Remember to listen to your body, make necessary adjustments to your fasting schedule, and consult with a healthcare professional if you experience persistent or severe side effects. With proper management, intermittent fasting can be a transformative and sustainable practice for optimal health and well-being.

CHAPTER 7: ADVANCED STRATEGIES FOR OPTIMAL HEALTH

Combining Intermittent Fasting with a Specific Diet

When it comes to optimizing your health through intermittent fasting, one of the most effective strategies is to combine it with a specific diet. While intermittent fasting alone can provide numerous benefits, pairing it with a well-balanced and nutrient-rich eating plan can supercharge your results and help you achieve your health goals faster.

There are several popular diets that work harmoniously with intermittent fasting, such as the ketogenic diet, the Mediterranean diet, and the paleo diet. Each of these diets has its unique approach to nutrition, but they all share the common goal of promoting overall health and well-being.

The ketogenic diet, for instance, is a low-carb, high-fat diet that forces your body to burn fat for fuel instead of carbohydrates. By following this diet while practicing intermittent fasting, you can accelerate your body's transition into a state of ketosis, where it becomes highly efficient at burning stored fat for energy. This combination is known to enhance weight loss, improve mental clarity, and increase energy levels.

On the other hand, the Mediterranean diet focuses on consuming whole foods, such as fruits, vegetables, whole grains, lean proteins, and healthy fats. It is rich in antioxidants, vitamins, and minerals, making it an excellent choice for those who want to improve their cardiovascular health, reduce inflammation, and maintain a healthy weight. When combined with intermittent fasting, the Mediterranean diet can help stabilize blood sugar levels and enhance the benefits of fasting.

The paleo diet, inspired by the eating habits of our ancestors, emphasizes consuming lean proteins, fruits, vegetables, nuts, and seeds while avoiding processed foods, grains, and dairy. When practiced alongside intermittent fasting, the paleo diet can lead to weight loss, increased muscle mass, improved digestion, and reduced inflammation.

It's important to remember that each person's dietary needs and preferences are unique. Therefore, it is crucial to consult with a healthcare professional or a registered dietitian before embarking on any specific diet while practicing intermittent fasting. They can help you determine which diet aligns best with your goals and provide personalized guidance to ensure you are meeting your nutritional needs.

Combining intermittent fasting with a specific diet can be a powerful tool in optimizing your health. Whether your aim is weight loss, improved cardiovascular health, increased energy levels, or overall well-being, finding the right diet to complement your intermittent fasting routine can amplify your results and help you achieve optimal health.

Intermittent Fasting for Athletes and Fitness Enthusiasts

In today's fast-paced world, more and more individuals are turning to intermittent fasting to improve their overall health and fitness levels. Athletes and fitness enthusiasts, in particular, can greatly benefit from incorporating this practice into their daily routine. In this subchapter, we will explore why intermittent fasting is not only compatible with an active lifestyle but can also enhance athletic performance and optimize fitness goals.

Intermittent fasting, also known as dynamic fasting, is a pattern of eating that involves alternating periods of fasting and eating within a specific time window. It has gained popularity due to its numerous health benefits, including weight loss, improved insulin sensitivity, increased energy levels, and enhanced mental clarity.

For athletes and fitness enthusiasts, intermittent fasting can provide an array of advantages. Firstly, it promotes fat burning and muscle preservation, which is crucial for those looking to improve body composition and performance. By extending the overnight fasting period and delaying breakfast, the body taps into stored fat as a source of fuel, leading to increased fat loss. Simultaneously, muscle mass is preserved and even potentially increased due to the release of human growth hormone (HGH) during fasting periods.

Moreover, intermittent fasting has been shown to improve cardiovascular health and boost endurance. Research suggests that fasting can enhance the body's ability to utilize stored fat as an energy source, sparing muscle glycogen for more extended physical activities. This metabolic adaptation can lead to improved endurance and sustained energy levels during workouts or competitions.

Additionally, intermittent fasting has been found to increase autophagy, a cellular cleaning process that removes damaged cells and proteins. This mechanism helps to reduce inflammation and promotes tissue repair, aiding in post-workout recovery and reducing the risk of injuries.

However, it is important to note that athletes and fitness enthusiasts must approach intermittent fasting with caution. Proper planning of fasting and eating windows is crucial to ensure adequate nutrient intake and fuel availability for optimal performance. It is recommended to consult with a healthcare professional or a registered dietitian who specializes in sports nutrition to develop an individualized fasting strategy that aligns with specific fitness goals and training schedules.

In conclusion, intermittent fasting can be a valuable tool for athletes and fitness enthusiasts seeking to enhance their performance, improve body composition, and optimize overall health. By incorporating this practice into their routine, individuals can experience the benefits of increased fat burning, improved endurance, and enhanced recovery. Nevertheless, it is essential to approach fasting with careful planning and guidance to ensure that nutritional needs are met, and performance is not compromised.

Intermittent Fasting for Mental Clarity and Cognitive Function

In the fast-paced world we live in today, maintaining mental clarity and cognitive function has become increasingly important. The constant bombardment of information and the pressure to multitask can leave our minds feeling overwhelmed and sluggish. But what if there was a simple and effective way to boost our mental clarity and enhance our cognitive function? Enter intermittent fasting.

Intermittent fasting, a practice that involves alternating periods of fasting and eating, has gained widespread popularity for its numerous health benefits. While most people associate intermittent fasting with weight loss and improved physical health, its impact on mental clarity and cognitive function is often overlooked.

One of the key mechanisms behind the mental benefits of intermittent fasting lies in the regulation of insulin levels. When we consume food, our bodies release insulin to help transport glucose into our cells for energy. However, when insulin levels remain constantly elevated due to frequent eating, it can lead to insulin resistance and inflammation, both of which can negatively impact brain health.

By practicing intermittent fasting, we give our bodies a break from the constant influx of food and allow insulin levels to stabilize.

This, in turn, promotes better insulin sensitivity and reduces inflammation, creating an optimal environment for improved mental clarity and cognitive function.

Additionally, intermittent fasting triggers a state of ketosis, where the body starts using stored fat as a source of energy instead of glucose. Ketones, the by-products of fat metabolism, have been shown to have neuroprotective effects and enhance brain function. This can result in improved focus, concentration, and overall mental performance.

Moreover, intermittent fasting has been found to increase the production of brain-derived neurotrophic factor (BDNF), a protein that supports the growth and survival of brain cells. Higher levels of BDNF have been associated with improved learning, memory, and mood regulation.

To harness the mental benefits of intermittent fasting, it is essential to adopt a structured fasting schedule and adhere to it consistently. There are various fasting protocols to choose from, such as the 16/8 method, where you fast for 16 hours and have an 8-hour eating window, or the 5:2 diet, where you eat normally for five days and restrict calories for two non-consecutive days.

In conclusion, intermittent fasting is not just a powerful tool for improving physical health and aiding weight loss; it also has profound effects on mental clarity and cognitive function. By regulating insulin levels, promoting ketosis, and increasing the production of BDNF, intermittent fasting can enhance focus, concentration, and overall brain performance. Whether you're a busy professional, a student, or simply looking to improve your mental acuity, incorporating intermittent fasting into your lifestyle may be the key to unlocking your full cognitive potential.

Intermittent Fasting for Longevity and Disease Prevention

In the fast-paced world we live in today, it's no surprise that many people are looking for effective ways to improve their health and longevity. One such method that has gained significant attention is intermittent fasting. This powerful practice has been proven to not only promote weight loss but also enhance overall health and prevent various diseases.

Intermittent fasting involves cycling between periods of fasting and eating. Unlike traditional diets that focus on what you eat, intermittent fasting focuses on when you eat. By restricting your eating window and giving your body a break from constant digestion, intermittent fasting allows your body to enter a state of autophagy, a natural cellular cleansing process that helps remove damaged cells and promote cellular regeneration.

Numerous studies have shown that intermittent fasting can have a profound impact on longevity and disease prevention. One key benefit is its ability to improve insulin sensitivity and regulate blood sugar levels. By giving your body a break from constant influxes of glucose, intermittent fasting can help reduce the risk of developing type 2 diabetes and improve overall metabolic health.

Additionally, intermittent fasting has been linked to a reduced risk of heart disease. It can lower blood pressure, improve cholesterol levels, and reduce inflammation, all of which are crucial factors in maintaining a healthy cardiovascular system. By incorporating intermittent fasting into your lifestyle, you can significantly reduce your risk of heart-related ailments and promote a longer, healthier life.

Furthermore, intermittent fasting has shown promising effects in preventing age-related cognitive decline. Studies have found that this practice can enhance brain function, improve memory, and protect against neurodegenerative diseases such as Alzheimer's and Parkinson's. By promoting the growth of new nerve cells and increasing the production of brain-derived neurotrophic factor (BDNF), intermittent fasting can help keep your brain sharp and resilient

It's important to note that intermittent fasting is not a one-size-fits-all approach. Each individual may have different needs and preferences when it comes to fasting protocols. It's essential to consult with a healthcare professional or a registered dietitian before embarking on an intermittent fasting journey, especially if you have any underlying medical conditions or are taking medication.

In conclusion, intermittent fasting is a powerful tool that can be utilized for both longevity and disease prevention. By incorporating this practice into your lifestyle, you can improve insulin sensitivity, reduce the risk of heart disease, and protect against age-related cognitive decline. However, it's crucial to approach intermittent fasting with caution and seek professional guidance to ensure it aligns with your unique needs and goals.

CHAPTER 8: MAINTAINING LONG-TERM SUCCESS WITH INTERMITTENT FASTING

Tracking and Monitoring Your Progress

One of the crucial aspects of mastering intermittent fasting is tracking and monitoring your progress. By keeping a close eye on your journey, you can better understand how your body responds to different fasting protocols and adjust accordingly for optimal results. Whether you are new to intermittent fasting or have been practicing it for a while, tracking and monitoring your progress will help you stay motivated and make informed decisions about your health.

Tracking your progress begins with setting clear and specific goals. Ask yourself why you are practicing intermittent fasting and what you hope to achieve. Are you looking to lose weight, improve your energy levels, or enhance your overall well-being? Once you have established your goals, you can track your progress towards them. Consider using a journal or a dedicated app to record your daily fasting schedule, the types of foods you consume during your eating window, and any physical or mental changes you experience.

Monitoring your progress involves paying attention to how your body responds to intermittent fasting. Keep an eye on your hunger levels, energy levels, and overall mood throughout the day. Are you feeling more alert and focused during your fasting period? Are you experiencing any cravings or energy dips? By observing these patterns, you can make adjustments to your fasting schedule or eating habits to better suit your body's needs.

Another important aspect of monitoring your progress is tracking your body measurements and weight. While the number on the scale is not the only indicator of progress, it can be a helpful tool to gauge changes in your body composition. Take regular measurements of your waist, hips, and other target areas to monitor changes in your body shape. Additionally, keep track of other markers of health such as blood pressure, cholesterol levels, and blood sugar levels to assess your overall well-being.

Remember that everyone's journey with intermittent fasting is unique. What works for one person may not work for another. By tracking and monitoring your progress, you can gain valuable insights into what works best for your body. Be patient with yourself and celebrate even the smallest victories along the way. With consistent tracking and monitoring, you will be able to optimize your intermittent fasting practice and achieve your health goals.

Adjusting Your Fasting Schedule as Needed

Intermittent fasting is a flexible and customizable approach to eating that can be adjusted to suit your individual needs and lifestyle. While there are many different fasting schedules to choose from, it is important to remember that what works for one person may not work for another. In order to truly master intermittent fasting and achieve optimal health, it is crucial to be open to adjusting your fasting schedule as needed.

One of the key principles of intermittent fasting is to listen to your body and honour its signals. This means paying attention to how you feel during your fasting periods and adjusting your schedule accordingly. For example, if you find that you are experiencing excessive hunger or low energy levels during a particular fasting window, it may be a sign that your body needs a different approach.

There are several ways to adjust your fasting schedule if you find it isn't working for you. One option is to experiment with different fasting windows. For example, if you have been following a 16:8 fasting schedule (fasting for 16 hours and eating within an 8-hour window) but find it difficult to sustain, you could try a 14:10 or even a 12:12 schedule instead. This allows for a shorter fasting period and may be more manageable for some individuals.

Another option is to consider alternate-day fasting or modified fasting. Alternate-day fasting involves fasting every other day, while modified fasting allows for a reduced-calorie intake on fasting days. These variations can provide more flexibility while still reaping the benefits of intermittent fasting.

It is also important to remember that intermittent fasting is not a one-size-fits-all approach. Factors such as age, gender, activity level, and overall health can influence your fasting experience. Therefore, it is essential to consult with a healthcare professional or registered dietitian before making any significant changes to your fasting schedule.

In conclusion, adjusting your fasting schedule as needed is a crucial part of mastering intermittent fasting. By being open to experimentation and listening to your body, you can find a fasting routine that works best for you. Remember to be patient and give yourself time to adapt to any new schedule. With practice and perseverance, you can achieve optimal health through dynamic fasting.

Strategies for Breaking a Fast

Breaking a fast is just as important as the fast itself. After a period of prolonged fasting, it is crucial to reintroduce food to your body in a gentle and mindful manner. This subchapter will provide you with essential strategies for breaking a fast effectively, ensuring optimal health benefits and a smooth transition back to regular eating.

1. Start with liquids: Begin by hydrating your body with water or herbal teas. This helps to rehydrate your system and prepare your digestive tract for food.
2. Incorporate light, easily digestible foods: Choose foods that are gentle on your digestive system, such as soups, broths, or smoothies. These foods are easier to break down and assimilate, allowing your body to adjust to the reintroduction of solid foods gradually.
3. . Focus on nutrient-dense foods: After a fast, your body is in a prime state to absorb nutrients. Opt for nutrient-dense foods like fruits, vegetables, lean proteins, and healthy fats. These foods will provide your body with essential vitamins, minerals, and antioxidants, supporting optimal health.
4. Chew your food thoroughly: Take the time to chew your food thoroughly before swallowing. Chewing properly aids digestion and allows your body to extract maximum nutrients from the food.
5. Listen to your body: Pay attention to your body's signals and eat until you feel satisfied, not overly full. Fasting helps improve your body's hunger and satiety cues, so trust your instincts and stop eating when you feel satisfied.
6. Avoid processed and sugary foods: While breaking a fast, it's crucial to avoid highly processed foods and those high in sugar. These foods can cause a spike in blood sugar levels and may lead to digestive discomfort or energy crashes.

7. Gradually reintroduce regular meals: Once you have successfully broken your fast, gradually transition back to regular eating patterns. Start with smaller, balanced meals and slowly increase portion sizes over a few days.

Remember, breaking a fast is a personal experience, and it may vary from person to person. It's essential to listen to your body's needs and adjust your approach accordingly. By following these strategies, you can ensure a smooth and beneficial transition from fasting to regular eating, supporting your overall health and well-being.

"Mastering Intermittent Fasting: Essential Practices for Optimal Health" provides detailed guidance on various fasting strategies, including dynamic fasting, aimed at anyone interested in harnessing the benefits of intermittent fasting for their health and well-being. Whether you are a beginner or experienced faster, this book will equip you with the knowledge and tools to master intermittent fasting and optimize your health.

Building Sustainable Habits for Lifelong Health

In today's fast-paced world, maintaining good health has become a priority for people from all walks of life. We all desire to live a long and fulfilling life, free from the burden of diseases and ailments that can hinder our well-being. One effective way to achieve optimal health is through the practice of intermittent fasting. In this subchapter, we will explore the essential practices for building sustainable habits that will support lifelong health.

Intermittent fasting is not just a diet; it is a lifestyle that promotes overall well-being by allowing the body to rest and rejuvenate. However, like any lifestyle change, it requires commitment and consistency. Here are some key practices to help you integrate intermittent fasting into your daily routine and make it a sustainable habit for lifelong health.

Firstly, it is crucial to start with small, achievable goals. Begin by incorporating shorter fasting periods into your routine and gradually increase the fasting window as your body adjusts. This approach will ensure a smooth transition and prevent any feelings of deprivation or overwhelm.

Secondly, it is essential to listen to your body. Pay attention to the signals it gives you during the fasting and eating periods. If you feel excessively hungry or fatigued, it may be a sign to adjust your fasting window or meal composition. Remember, intermittent fasting is a flexible practice that can be tailored to suit your individual needs.

Next, focus on nourishing your body with nutrient-dense foods during your eating window. Intermittent fasting is not an excuse to indulge in unhealthy eating habits. Make a conscious effort to include a variety of fruits, vegetables, lean proteins, and whole grains in your meals. This will provide your body with the necessary nutrients for optimal health.

In addition to a balanced diet, regular physical activity is crucial for lifelong health. Incorporate exercise into your routine, whether it is a brisk walk, yoga, or strength training. Exercise not only aids in weight management but also improves cardiovascular health, enhances mental well-being, and boosts overall energy levels.

Lastly, surround yourself with a supportive community. Building sustainable habits is easier when you have like-minded individuals to share your journey with. Join online forums, attend local meetups, or form a small group of friends who are also interested in intermittent fasting. Share your experiences, seek advice, and motivate each other to stay on track.

By incorporating these essential practices into your daily life, you will be well on your way to building sustainable habits for lifelong health through intermittent fasting. Remember, it is a journey, and progress is more important than perfection. Stay committed, be patient with yourself, and embrace the transformative power of intermittent fasting.

CHAPTER 9: FREQUENTLY ASKED QUESTIONS ABOUT INTERMITTENT FASTING

Can I Drink Coffee or Tea During Fasting Hours?

One of the most common questions that arise when starting intermittent fasting is whether or not you can drink coffee or tea during fasting hours. The answer to this question largely depends on the type of fasting protocol you are following and your personal goals.

If you are following the dynamic fasting approach to intermittent fasting, where you cycle between periods of fasting and eating throughout the day, then consuming coffee or tea during fasting hours is generally acceptable. Both coffee and tea are low in calories and can provide a boost of energy and mental clarity, which can be especially beneficial during fasting periods when you may experience some hunger or fatigue.

However, it is important to note that you should drink your coffee or tea without any added sugars, creamers, or milk. These additions can break your fast and spike your insulin levels, which can disrupt the metabolic benefits of fasting. Instead, opt for black coffee or unsweetened herbal teas to keep your body in a fasting state.

Coffee, in particular, has been shown to have numerous health benefits when consumed in moderation. It contains antioxidants and caffeine, which can help improve mental focus, boost metabolism, and even enhance fat burning during fasting periods. Additionally, coffee has been linked to a reduced risk of certain diseases, such as type 2 diabetes and Parkinson's disease.

Tea, on the other hand, offers a wide range of health benefits as well. It is rich in antioxidants and can promote relaxation, improve digestion, and support immune function. Green tea, in particular, has been shown to boost metabolism and aid in weight loss, making it a great choice for those practicing intermittent fasting for weight management.

Ultimately, the decision to drink coffee or tea during fasting hours is up to you and should be based on your personal preferences and goals. If you find that it helps you stay focused and energized during fasting periods, then go ahead and enjoy a cup or two. Just remember to keep it black or unsweetened to maximize the benefits of fasting.

In conclusion, drinking coffee or tea during fasting hours is generally acceptable, especially if you are following the dynamic fasting approach. Both beverages can provide a boost of energy and mental clarity without significantly impacting your fasting state. Just be sure to avoid adding any sugars, creamers, or milk to keep your body in a fasting state and reap the maximum benefits of intermittent fasting.

Is Intermittent Fasting Safe for Everyone?

Intermittent fasting has gained significant popularity in recent years as a powerful tool for weight loss and overall health improvement. However, many people wonder if this eating pattern is safe for everyone. In this subchapter, we will explore the safety of intermittent fasting and discuss who should approach it with caution.

First and foremost, it is important to note that intermittent fasting is generally considered safe for most healthy individuals. It can be an effective strategy for weight loss, insulin sensitivity, and reducing inflammation. However, it may not be suitable for everyone, especially those with certain medical conditions or specific dietary needs.

Pregnant or breastfeeding women should avoid intermittent fasting, as they have increased nutrient requirements to support the growth and development of their baby. Fasting during this crucial period may deprive both the mother and the baby of essential nutrients, potentially leading to complications.

Similarly, individuals with a history of disordered eating should approach intermittent fasting with caution. Restricting food intake may trigger unhealthy behaviours or feelings of deprivation, which can exacerbate the underlying psychological issues. It is essential for those with disordered eating patterns to seek professional guidance before embarking on any fasting regimen.

People with diabetes or other chronic medical conditions should also consult their healthcare provider before starting intermittent fasting. Fasting can affect blood sugar levels, and adjustments to medication or insulin dosage may be necessary to prevent any adverse effects. Close monitoring and guidance from a healthcare professional are crucial to ensure safety and optimize health outcomes.

It is worth mentioning that intermittent fasting may not be suitable for children and teenagers, as they require a well-balanced diet to support their growth and development. Fasting during these critical stages of life may hinder proper nutrient intake and potentially impact their overall health.

In summary, while intermittent fasting can offer numerous health benefits for most individuals, it is not suitable for everyone. Pregnant or breastfeeding women, individuals with a history of disordered eating, those with chronic medical conditions, and children or teenagers should exercise caution and seek professional advice before adopting an intermittent fasting regimen. By prioritizing safety and individual needs, one can make informed decisions about incorporating intermittent fasting into their lifestyle and reap the benefits it has to offer.

Can I Take Medications or Supplements While Fasting?

When it comes to intermittent fasting, one of the common concerns people have is whether they can take medications or supplements while fasting. This subchapter aims to address this question and provide guidance for anyone practicing dynamic fasting.

The short answer is yes, you can take medications or supplements while fasting. However, there are a few important considerations to keep in mind. It's crucial to consult with your healthcare provider before making any changes to your medication routine or starting any new supplements, especially if you have underlying health conditions.

Medications: If you have prescribed medications that need to be taken regularly, it's generally recommended to continue taking them as prescribed, even during fasting periods. Medications such as blood pressure medications, insulin, or thyroid medications should not be skipped or altered without medical advice. Remember, the primary goal of intermittent fasting is to promote overall health and well-being, and you should never compromise your health for the sake of fasting.

Supplements: While taking supplements during fasting is generally allowed, it's important to choose wisely. Some supplements may contain calories or artificial sweeteners, which can break your fast. Opt for supplements that are specifically designed for fasting, such as electrolytes, vitamins, or minerals. These supplements can support your overall health and replenish any potential deficiencies that may arise during fasting.

However, it's crucial to note that some supplements, particularly fat-soluble vitamins, may require fat intake for optimal absorption. In such cases, it's recommended to take these supplements with a small amount of healthy fat, such as a teaspoon of olive oil or a handful of nuts, to ensure proper absorption.

In conclusion, while taking medications or supplements during fasting is generally acceptable, it's essential to prioritize your health and consult with your healthcare provider. They will provide you with personalized advice based on your specific medical needs. Remember, intermittent fasting is a tool for improving health, and it should never compromise your well-being or medical treatment.

Continue reading "Mastering Intermittent Fasting: Essential Practices for Optimal Health" to learn more about dynamic fasting and its essential practices for achieving optimal health.

How Does Intermittent Fasting Impact Women's Health?

Intermittent fasting has gained significant popularity in recent years as a powerful tool for improving overall health and well-being. However, many women wonder whether this eating pattern is suitable for them and how it may affect their specific health needs. In this subchapter, we will explore the impact of intermittent fasting on women's health, addressing common concerns and providing essential practices for optimal well-being.

One of the primary concerns women have regarding intermittent fasting is its potential impact on hormonal balance. Hormones play a crucial role in women's health, regulating menstrual cycles, fertility, and overall mood. While intermittent fasting can have positive effects on hormonal balance, it is essential to approach it with care. Women should consider adjusting their fasting schedule to align with their menstrual cycle, as fasting during the luteal phase may be more challenging due to increased hunger and cravings. Additionally, ensuring adequate nutrition during the eating window is crucial to support hormonal health and prevent any potential disruptions.

Another area of concern is the impact of intermittent fasting on fertility. While research in this specific area is still limited, there is evidence to suggest that intermittent fasting can improve fertility by reducing insulin resistance and supporting healthy weight management. However, it is crucial for women who are trying to conceive to consult with their healthcare provider before implementing an intermittent fasting regimen, as individual circumstances may vary.

Weight management is another aspect of women's health that can be positively influenced by intermittent fasting. Studies have shown that intermittent fasting can be an effective strategy for weight loss, as it helps to reduce overall calorie intake and improve metabolic function. However, it is important to approach weight management with a balanced mindset and focus on overall health rather than solely on appearance

Furthermore, intermittent fasting has been associated with various benefits for women's health, such as improved insulin sensitivity, reduced inflammation, and enhanced brain function. By giving the body regular periods of rest from food, intermittent fasting allows it to focus on repair and rejuvenation, leading to improved overall health and vitality.

In conclusion, intermittent fasting can have a significant impact on women's health when approached with care and consideration for individual needs. By adjusting the fasting schedule according to the menstrual cycle, ensuring adequate nutrition, and seeking guidance from healthcare providers, women can harness the benefits of intermittent fasting to optimize their well-being. Whether it is for hormonal balance, fertility, weight management, or overall health, mastering intermittent fasting can be a valuable practice for women of all ages and backgrounds.

CHAPTER 10: CONCLUSION: EMBRACING A HEALTHIER LIFESTYLE WITH INTERMITTENT FASTING

Congratulations! You have reached the end of our journey together in exploring the world of intermittent fasting. Throughout this book, we have delved into the essential practices and principles that can help you achieve optimal health through intermittent fasting. As we conclude this chapter, let us recap the key takeaways and encourage you to embrace a healthier lifestyle with intermittent fasting.

Intermittent fasting, or dynamic fasting as we have explored it, is not just another diet fad. It is a powerful tool that can transform your life by promoting weight loss, improving metabolic health, increasing mental clarity, and even extending your lifespan. The flexibility and simplicity of intermittent fasting make it accessible to anyone, regardless of their lifestyle or dietary preferences.

By adopting dynamic fasting, you can train your body to tap into its fat stores for energy during fasting periods, leading to significant weight loss and improved body composition.

Moreover, intermittent fasting has been shown to promote autophagy, a process of cellular rejuvenation that can have anti-aging effects and reduce the risk of chronic diseases.

Throughout this book, we have discussed the various methods of intermittent fasting, such as the 16/8 method, the 5:2 diet, and alternate-day fasting. Each approach has its unique benefits and can be tailored to suit your individual needs and goals. Experimenting with different fasting protocols can help you find the one that fits seamlessly into your lifestyle.

However, it is important to remember that intermittent fasting is not a one-size-fits-all solution. It may not be suitable for everyone, especially those with certain medical conditions or nutritional needs. Before embarking on any fasting regimen, it is crucial to consult with a healthcare professional who can guide you through the process and ensure your safety.

In conclusion, intermittent fasting is a practice that can revolutionize your health and well-being. By embracing a healthier lifestyle with intermittent fasting, you can achieve weight management, enhance your metabolism, and improve your overall health. Remember to start slowly, listen to your body, and make adjustments along the way. With dedication and consistency, intermittent fasting can become a sustainable and rewarding part of your life, allowing you to unlock the full potential of your body and mind.

Thank you for joining us on this journey, and we wish you all the best in your pursuit of optimal health through intermittent fasting!